THE WAY OF THE 4TH TOE

Also by Jack Wiener

Creative Movement for Children: A Dance Program for the Classroom
Article: "Silence Is Depression's Glue" for Crisis magazine (NAACP)

THE WAY OF THE 4TH TOE

Into the
Feeling Body

*Three simple adjustments
that profoundly alter the way stress
happens in the body*

Jack Wiener, Lp, Cdmt

iUniverse, Inc.
Bloomington

THE WAY OF THE 4TH TOE
Into the Feeling Body

iUniverse books may be ordered through booksellers or by contacting:

iUniverse
1663 Liberty Drive
Bloomington, IN 47403
www.iuniverse.com
1-800-Authors (1-800-288-4677)

ISBN: 978-1-4620-2780-4 (sc)
ISBN: 978-1-4620-2781-1 (ebk)

Printed in the United States of America

iUniverse rev. date: 09/20/2011

For my children, Josh and Rama,
and my grandchildren,
Nathaniel, Aden, and Kika

John: *What do you think is the greatest thing that dance has taught you? What is the real secret—that it has given you?*

Jeffrey: **Feeling—the whole secret is** *feeling.*

John: *Do you want to explain that a little more, Jeff?*

Jeffrey: **Well—it's hard to explain because everybody has a different feeling. With myself—I just feel new, I feel . . . fresh. I'm a new person, like a newborn baby who just came out of the mother's body.**

John: *Each time you dance, Jeff?*

Jeffrey: **Each time.**

Excerpt from a taped conversation: Jeffrey Kern, age seven, with John Lidstone, Ed.D., director of Queens Youth Center for the Arts, Kew Gardens, New York City (1960); former dean, art education department, Queens College CUNY.

Appeared originally in
Creative Movement for Children:
A Dance Program for the Classroom
by Jack Wiener and John Lidstone

ACKNOWLEDGMENTS

I have to thank the hundreds of students who have shared their improvisations, teaching me to observe and understand how feelings come through in movement.

A special thanks to Gwen Barrows, a very wise ex-student and friend, who years ago suggested calling my book *The Way of the Fourth Toe*. I have to single out two people: Gus Sperber, a psychotherapist, whose emotional focus released an inner tension that led me to the physical parallel of *body weight and its channeling through the muscles*; and Elizabeth Thorne, my psychoanalyst, whose uncompromising pursuit of my primal defense opened my perception to how affects connect us internally, which led to the concept of the interplay of muscles. Her persistence, exhilarating and painful, made clear the difference between meanings, problem solving, and feeling.

My gratitude to Meg Chang, EdD, LCAT, NCC, BC-DMT, an internationally renowned dance therapist and longtime student, whose suggestions helped to format the material in a more accessible manner.

To Debra Bernath, NYLMT, reflexologist, qigong meridian therapist, and botanical illustrator, my appreciation for the exacting drawings.

Most of all to my wife, Arlette, whose careful readings over the years have helped me to be aware that I am sharing my heart, not just my mind. I hope that what I have learned from her will reach the reader of this journey.

Jack Wiener

ILLUSTRATIONS

BY DEBRA BERNATH

PREFACE

The muscles tighten to keep out the unwanted outside and unwanted inside. But they also loosen to let the desired outside in—and to let the inside flower!

When the muscles tighten, the flow of blood, which they help to pump throughout the body, decreases; when muscles loosen, the blood fills the heart and brain.

The secrets that the tight muscles hold affect our bodies and our minds. Opening the pathway of the muscles creates a safe road for the secrets to travel on.

This is the journey that I hope you will take with me by *The Way of the Fourth Toe: Into the Feeling Body*.

CONTENTS

QUALIFICATIONS FOR THE FEELING BODY

My journey into movement started with an artistic commitment to express an inner passion for which I could not find words.

I studied modern dance with its principal innovators: José Limón; Martha Graham; Alwin Nickolais and partner Murray Louis, who extended the work of Hanya Holm and Gertrud Kraus; and with Merce Cunningham, whose choreographic approach opened the gates for what is now current in the field. I also studied the Lester Horton technique with Jimmy Truitte at the Ninety-Second Street Y, in a class with Carmen de Lavallade and Alvin Ailey, whose celebrity as dancers and choreographers is well known to the general public. My ballet training was with Alfredo Corvino and the psychologically astute ballet choreographer Antony Tudor at Juilliard, where I was introduced to Rudolf Laban and labanotation, the most used system of dance recording and a theoretical basis for much of dance therapy, with one of its master proponents, Ann Hutchinson. I undertook additional ballet training with Julia Barashkova, a product of the incomparable Kirov school of St. Petersburg, Russia, from which Mikhail Baryshnikov emerged. Studies in composition were with Doris Humphrey, Louis Horst, and Lucas Hoving, whose names are etched in the pantheon of modern dance.

I danced with Charles Weidman of Humphrey-Weidman fame, and spent three years with the Fred Berk Company, which performed pieces by notable modern dance choreographers like Sophie Maslow, Alvin Ailey, and Jeff Duncan, a principal founder of the institutional Dance Theater Workshop. I auditioned and made the cut for the film version of *West Side Story*, with Jerome Robbins deciding who was in and who was out. There were also sundry classes in jazz and Afro-Cuban techniques.

Those were five intensive years of dancing seven to twelve hours a day.

When I began, muscles were simply to be made flexible and strong to fulfill the demands of professional dance and choreographic styles.

I taught the way I was taught by repeating dance steps and phrases of movement, with the implicit expectation that body memory would kick in. However, the vast majority of adult students in my classes were nonprofessionals for whom teaching the usual combinations of steps and gestures of arms and legs needed to be simplified. Given my high school engineering background, breaking things down to a one-two-three level came easily.

Discovering how difficult imitation was for my non-professional students, I abandoned steps and instead explored improvisational foci that opened up breathing, motion, beat, gesture, directions, impulses, space, and time—elements that are usually enmeshed in traditional training techniques. This exploratory approach satisfied the sense of dance as freedom and overcame inhibitions and judgments of right and wrong.

These explorations, which got students to move comfortably with all music, culminated in a seven-year syllabus designed for a range of students from beginners to more advanced dancers. Some students have been with me for close to forty years.

Although the improvisational approach liberated the cry for release and stimulated the imagination of educated, gifted, and accomplished adults, it lacked both physical and emotional definition. What was imagined in the head was not coming through the musculature.

It took twenty-five years of teaching before I began to see clearly how the muscles must be worked with to make the body truly present, given the overwhelming tendency of the mind to organize—interpret the experience of movement.

This book begins with what I finally discovered, *the interplay of muscles*. It begins with the three simple adjustments that absolutely everyone can manage. It leads eventually to an un–self-conscious emotional flow of our naturally endowed *feeling body*.

INTRODUCTION

How I got to *The Way of the Fourth Toe* is not only my journey; it is, I believe, everyone's path.

There are several layers to this book: telling you exactly what to try to do; describing ways of experiencing the body and movement for those of you who are dance students, professional dancers, lovers of movement; and talking to psychoanalysts and others who think seriously about the body and why we subordinate—even denigrate—it as regressive, in contrast to the cognitive mind.

You will recognize ways of perceiving your movement that contribute to physical and emotional problems. You will become aware of how the body reflexively defends against the natural flow of feelings that result in mixed messages that are different from the way we intend. And finally, I will show you how to make practical, incremental changes, regardless of what kind of physical activity or practice you engage in, that will alter lifelong, habitually aggravating patterns of posture and motion.

What is most surprising about this process is how it allows your deepest, most unconscious feelings to emerge as you tap into the way the psyche travels through the interplay of muscles.

That such a profound flow happens through muscular togetherness, with such a wide variety of adults (some who began with quite serious physical impediments), convinced me that this process does not hinge on skill or love of motion. It continually astonishes me.

How far you can take the process of the *interplay of muscles* depends on your commitment. I can assure you that every step of the way will be a move toward a healthier moving body, a surprising aliveness, and a simplicity of being that you will find hard to believe.

THE GROUND, THE EARTH

You stand on your feet and experience the sensation of contact to the floor rising up through the muscles of the feet, continuing up the musculature of the body all the way into the muscles of the neck. That's all there is to *the interplay of muscles—the feeling body*.

Everything we need for the feeling body is totally available: the ground to stand on, the soles of the feet that sense the contact to the earth, the nerves embedded in the muscles that carry the sensation to the brain, and the nerves that carry the messages back for movement. Nature has endowed us with the essentials needed for the deepest, most profound awareness of emotional aliveness, *because all feelings register through the body first*, before they become actions or thoughts or words.

Gestures, words, thoughts, ideas, concepts, and theories are discovered, learned, and created as we grow to relate physically and emotionally to ourselves and to others. The simplicity of physical aliveness recedes as the focus shifts to the pride of thinking and relating.

The remarkable thing about the musculature is that it continues working, regardless of whether or not we pay attention. Empathy, for example, has a physical sensibility. We sense in our bodies how another person might be feeling.

When we function as if attention to this muscular sensitivity isn't necessary, we dismiss how the body feeds our humanity. When gratifying others and self overshadows our physical constancy, we avoid our feelings. We tend to lose ourselves in acquiring control and mastery. We denigrate the body as hungry. Food and touch are unquestionably necessary for our survival as infants. However, the emotional connections to these needs too often remain unchanged. Many never shake off the hunger for food and for control of self and others. The habit for more, for getting filled, shows up literally

1

in obesity and symbolically in greed, in devouring relationships, in obstinate politics, in so many different aspects of our lives and personalities that continually negate the simplicity of our natural endowment for awareness of feelings.

Touch has been shown to be essential for the infant's sense of care and peace. Care and peace is what I believe meditation, in its many guises over thousands of years, has tried to do.

Through my fifty years of teaching, I have discovered how to engage this underlying profound process by the way of the fourth-toe-line contact with the ground and through the interplay of muscles.

FOR ANYONE AT ANY TIME: JUST DO IT!

THE THREE BASIC ADJUSTMENTS

Na'aseh v'nishma.
(We will do and we will hear.)

Exodus 24:7

1.) Stand over the fourth-toe line of the sole of the feet.

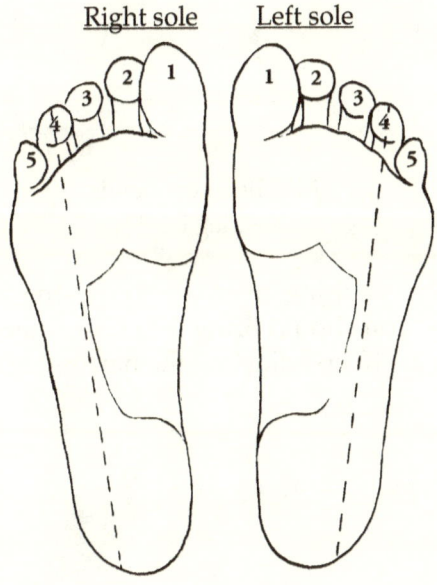

Right sole   Left sole

Take a number of steps forward, making sure to step over the fourth-toe line.

2.) Narrow your stance to make sure to step over the fourth-toe line.

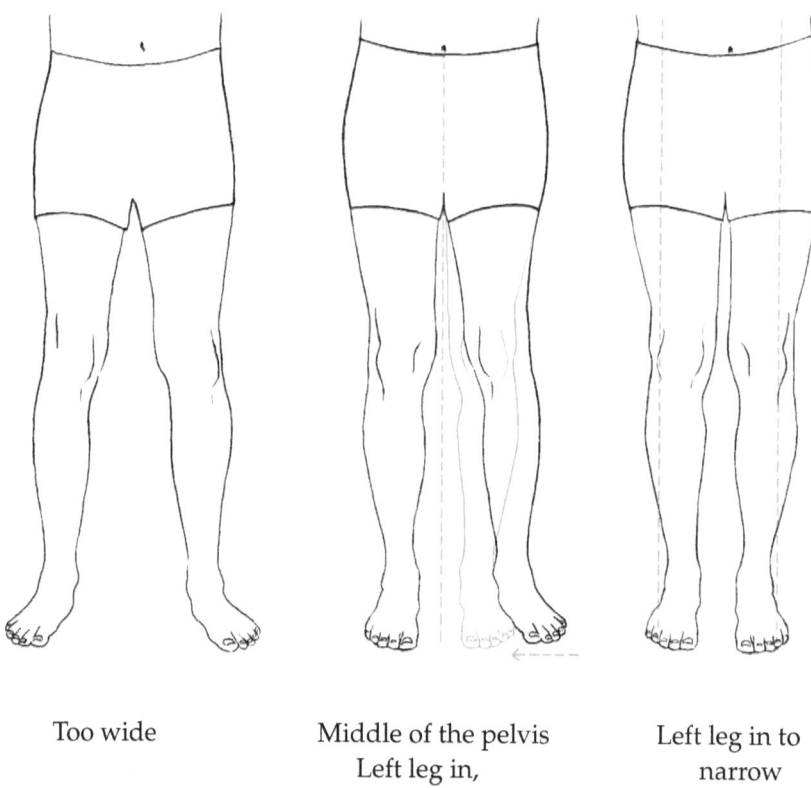

Too wide   Middle of the pelvis   Left leg in to
                      Left leg in,   narrow

The leg on which stepping over the fourth-toe line seems most unclear is the one you should bring into the center of your body to narrow your stance. Keep adjusting the narrowing until it feels just right.

3.) Shorten your stride to consistently step over the fourth-toe line of your feet as you walk, until the stride is just right.

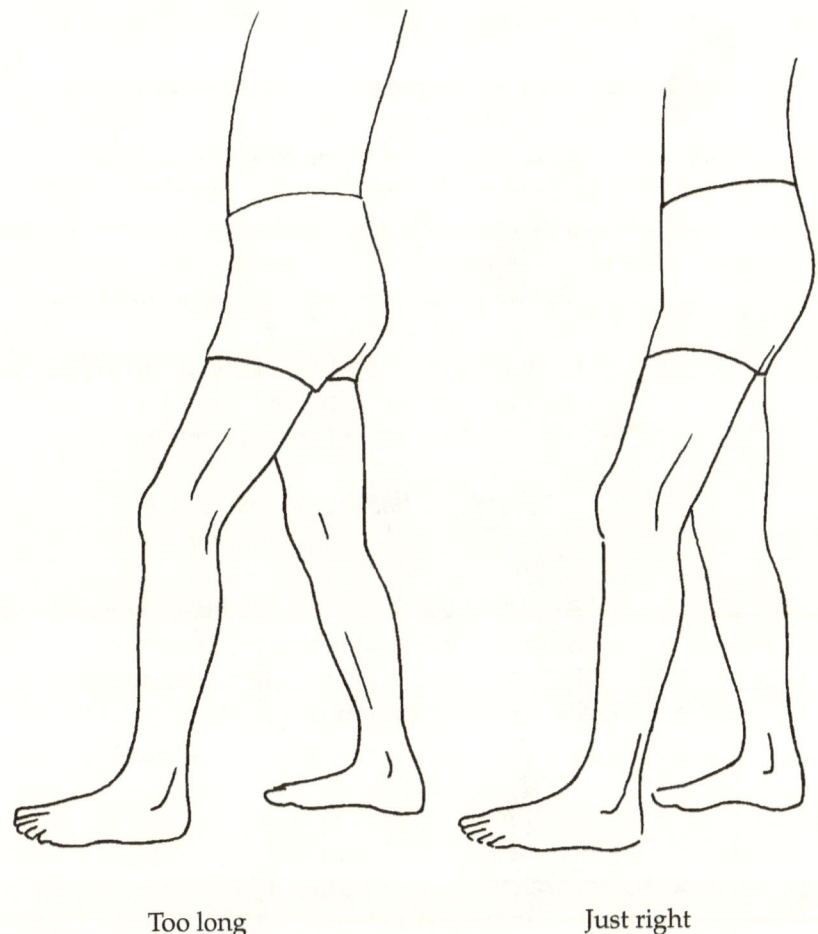

Too long   Just right

These three fundamental small adjustments will, over time, alter muscular misalignments from the feet all the way up through the neck, as the ground becomes your basic support. Upper body tension will melt away as the motion of movement goes around joints.

Anyone, at any time, can put these simple adjustments into play.

MAKING SURE OF THE FOURTH-TOE LINE

— *Sitting*

Sit on a straight-back chair barefooted. Raise your right heel, keeping your toes on the floor.

Bring your heel down while pressing down on your big toe.

You'll notice as you press down on the big toe that the ankle pushes inward, collapsing the arch and stressing the inside of the knee.

Do exactly the same heel lift, pressing down on the second toe, the arch still collapses, although slightly less. The knee is still stressed.

Do the same over the third toe; this collapses the arch even less.

Repeating the process over the fourth toe allows you to realize that it is the one line of the foot that *does not* collapse the arch at all, but supports it.

The fourth-toe line provides the most solid placement of the foot's contact with the floor.

Applying pressure over the little toe twists the ankle, giving the least solidity with the floor.

Repeating this whole sequence a few times will clarify your perceptions of what happened the first time.

Try the same process with your left foot.

By doing this exercise slowly, you will begin to sense that the fourth-toe line's contact with the floor is clearer with one foot.

If this is the case, you should bring the leg with the more insecure contact to the floor closer to the other leg, narrowing your stance.

Incrementally, bring the weaker contact leg closer to the more solid foot until the sensation with both feet feels totally the same.

There are many muscles that need to change in relationship to each other, which is why you must make the suggested changes incrementally.

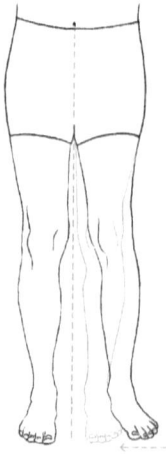

You may find it necessary to incrementally swivel the toes of one of the feet in toward the center of your body to sense the fourth-toe line on the sole of that foot more clearly. You may have to toe in slightly with both feet. It is not unusual for one foot to toe in more than the other. *Do not move your heels as you swivel your toes.*

Contact with both feet is very important in developing your ability to sense *symmetry of sensation*. The sensitivity to the symmetry of sensation will serve you as the corrective standard as you increasingly sense the compensatory misalignments that your body has patterned unconsciously. (Note that the need to make incremental adjustments in order to sense symmetry applies to all exercises.)

What you are learning is your *perception of motion through the muscles* and how to go about adjusting for a clearer flow of movement.

This sensitivity to the motion through the muscles will put you in charge of realigning your musculature in a very specific, personal way for which there is no substitute.

However much you incrementally adjust keeps adding to your sense of solidity coming *from the floor* rather than from holding your spine, shoulders, and neck in and up.

This is the beginning of altering patterns that have contributed to weak arches, tight ankles, scary sensations in your knees, hip pain, and lower back problems. You are simultaneously changing the physical patterns of the psychological repression of feelings, which involves the unconscious tightening of muscles and joints!

By repeating this simple process a number of times, the fourth-toe line on the sole of the feet will become irrefutable.

Remember that your brain is registering the solid support of contact, releasing the braced tension of overly contracted muscles throughout your entire body.

— Standing

Try to stand, maintaining the fourth-toe-line contact with the floor.

In the effort to stand up from a sitting position, you may find that either your knees come in toward each other as you push inward toward your groin, causing the ankles to press down and collapsing the arches, *or* you spread your knees out, maintaining a better fourth-toe-line contact while still pushing into the groin and overarching your lower back.

Although, in my experience, the knees coming in toward each other is more common, they both result from the habit of lifting the head upward to begin the movement of standing—a pattern going back to infancy when there was no other choice.

Our head and eyes telegraph our direction. We want to see where we are going, which sounds perfectly reasonable, except for the fact that it tends to overlook the constancy of our connection with the ground. Although toddlers are dependent on the ground, they are already focused on their intentions, control of their movement. They unconsciously negate the ground that supports them. Control already overwhelms what is actually happening to fulfill their intentions.

This unconscious suppression is so reflexive that it may shock you to realize what you have been doing all along without any awareness of it.

Is it any wonder that over the course of years, foot, knee, lower back, and neck problems are so prevalent? There is something self-destructive in this negation, or I should say, this *repression of kinesthetic awareness*.

Developing the awareness of standing over the fourth-toe-line contact to the earth begins to eliminate the physical, somatic expression of this unconscious self-destructive pattern.

— A New Way to Stand

Rising on top of the fourth-toe line to not collapse the arches, even minimally, predicates that you lean forward with your whole torso, letting your head hang down, which stretches your back and allows you to rise up, pushing into the floor through the fullness of the whole line of contact with the floor.

✦ A Case in Point ✦

Sarah had suffered a stroke affecting her left side and was diagnosed pre-Alzheimer. The stroke was a terrible blow to her characteristic independence, a trait that was already obvious by the time she was three years old. The stubbornness of her independence was manifested in an extremely stiff neck. In trying to get her to push off her contact with the floor, I had to hold her neck down over a number of weeks, increasing the pressure over time. She wanted to stand by lifting her head first, which made her knees go in toward each other, which in turn pushed the pelvis back, thereby weakening her lower back by making it curve into a lordosis. As she stood by pushing off the fourth line of her feet, her walking became increasingly more secure; and surprisingly, her pre-Alzheimer symptoms disappeared, as more blood entered her brain.

The solidity of your feet and the strength in your legs that you will begin to feel in rising to a standing position in this new way should be unquestionable.

The infantile pattern of leading with your head to come off the floor will finally disappear into your memory, rather than remaining an unconscious physical talisman of your determination.

It is shocking to realize how habits that are no longer necessary linger on in the body, creating unnecessary pressures that accompany the efforts of what we do!

I hope that this realization will convince you of how psychological most of these unnecessary habits embedded in the musculature are. The habits serve to obscure the feeling experience of what is currently happening. The mind replaces, by explanations and metaphors, the physicality of feelings—the ground of empathy.

By repeating and reminding yourself to stand in this new way until it is un–self-conscious, you will continually sense the changes throughout all the troubled spots in your body—areas that have been split off from the interplay of muscles, overly burdened again and again to hold you up.

It is the safety of the ground, the contact of our feet, and the sensation of the contact moving up through our muscles that fulfills our intentions. It is not our conceit that holds us up!

The sensitivity to the physical process accompanies the motivation that puts you more in touch simultaneously with what you are feeling.

I know from experience how we have to be reminded endlessly about habits before we can change them. *But it isn't hard to change if we remain aware.*

What makes changing muscular habits seem difficult is the wish for things to happen intuitively, the way we came to believe they happened when we were infants. Back then, process didn't register consciously, although it was clearly going on!

What should be obvious is that standing over the fourth-toe line of the sole of the foot is only the start of sensing through the musculature. It is a concrete sensation that is not mutually exclusive from any other framework by which we look to understand our actions. It is the experience of doing that counts!

— *Walking*

Take a step forward and see if you can step over the fourth-toe line of the foot.

You may find it easy if you are being very careful. However, most people immediately realize that their stride is usually too big, making it difficult to continually step over the fourth-toe line.

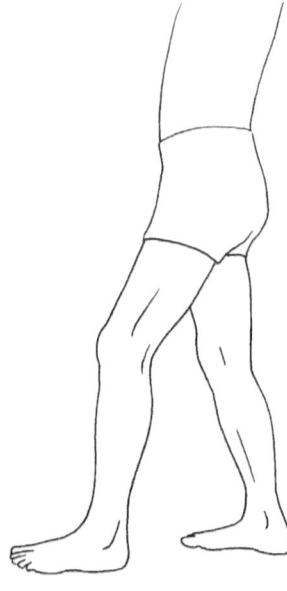

- The obvious correction is to shorten your stride.
- Do this *incrementally* until your stride is just right!
- The *just-right stride* is neither too long nor too short.
- The just-right stride allows for always stepping over the fourth-toe line.

Too long

The just-right stride varies depending on the length of your legs and how wide or narrow the distance between your legs is.

If the distance between your legs is too wide, you may experience shortening your stride as curtailing the force of your motivation. If your stance is too narrow, you may experience stepping over the fourth-toe line as taking baby steps.

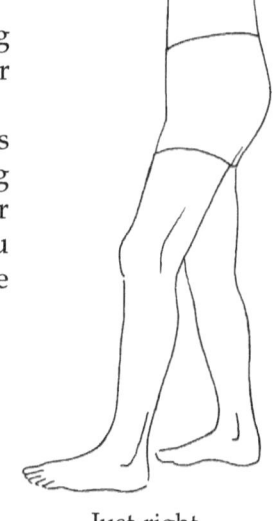

Just-right

By narrowing your stance (reducing the distance between your legs), you will find it much easier to step over the fourth-toe line.

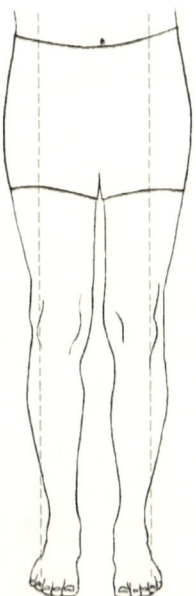

Both the narrowing of your stance and the shortening of your stride must be done incrementally, until it feels just right.

Far too many people have a stance that is more in keeping with the width of their hips, rather than the musculature through which motion happens. The connection to the width of the hips is psychological, a sense of growing up. Skeletal alignment *does not guarantee* the clear functioning of the musculature through which movement happens.

Narrowing the stance and shortening the stride facilitate a commensurate interplay of muscles rising from the fourth-toe line through the feet, into the outside of the calves, around the knees, and into the perineum, aligning the pelvis under the torso and allowing the motion of walking to fully, not partially, transfer the weight through the musculature.

Just-right stance

No other correction that I know of compares with these three simple adjustments—adjustments that we are all equipped to make.

REVIEW

- Find the solid contact of the fourth-toe line on the sole of the feet.
- Rise to a standing position on the fourth-toe line contact.
- Shorten your stride as you walk, to step clearly over the fourth-toe line.
- Narrow your stance to channel the motion through the muscles.

If you can become totally alive to these three incremental adjustments, you will have the basis for staying in your body as you do whatever you do. It is the essence of all the adjustments which subsequent sections of the book make clear, that lead into the feeling body.

HOW DO YOU EXPERIENCE YOUR BODY?

Before going into the specifics of how to exercise more personally and self-protectively, as a follow-through from the previous section, I'd like to ask you to consider how you think about and experience your body. It makes a big difference in the way you will make use of the ground, the fourth line of the feet, narrowing your stance, and shortening your stride.

In the fifty-some years of teaching, I've differentiated three relatively distinctive body-movement personalities. One of them should more or less fit you.

THREE PERSONALITY TYPES

Is your body a tool to be used, coordinated, and mastered? Or is your body an organism, full of sensations to be monitored, verging on pain or prone to accidents? Or is your body a channel for messages alerting you to something around you or premonitions within? Each is a unique universe to be understood and appreciated.

Each way of thinking about your body affects the way you perceive the extension of an arm; experience motion through space and the fullness or emptiness of the body; sense whether an impulse insists on expulsion or suppression; and respond to music or another person. Each also affects whether you sense your gestures expressing or containing what you are feeling.

The perceptions of the body as a tool and an organism are pretty common. The concept of the body as a channel may seem esoteric, but not to the artist, the mystic, or the doctor for whom physical signals are messages coming through the body!

Which one of these do you identify with?

THE BODY AS A TOOL

— *A Personal Example*

When I played football as an adolescent, without shoulder pads or a helmet, it became obvious to me that I needed to tackle low around the knees and ankles to bring the runner down; otherwise, I would just bounce off my friends' bodies, given their size and speed. I also realized that, because of the size of my hands, I needed to grip the football closer to the end to spiral my throw. I naturally used my body as a tool that helped me to *master* the activity I was involved in. It was a body I was proud to *control*.

As kids, we all figured out how to do things in relationship to our size, speed, and strength. We imitated the kids who were older or better than us and adjusted our skills accordingly. It seemed to me that everyone thought alike. If you didn't figure out how to adjust, chances were that you just dropped that particular physical activity. I was doing for myself what I later came to realize most teaching and coaching approaches do: someone shows, and we imitate. I call this "the body as a tool."

— *Dance Training*

Most dance training: ballet, modern, Afro-Cuban, Indian, Balinese, and so on, follows this imitative approach. The teacher demonstrates the movement, and the student follows. It is mostly a nonverbal tradition, not unlike how an infant absorbs during the early weeks, months, and years of life![1]

Dancing is a relatively silent art environment in which understanding through imitation is standard and expected.

We are loved and encouraged by parents in the mastery and control of the body. This is true, with variations, everywhere in the world. The body as a tool is the most prevalent of all the perspectives about the body.

— *Love and Imitation!*

When my granddaughter, just shy of two years old at the time, imitated her father's playful question, *"Wha'chu'du'en?"* the imitation was perfect: the words, the contraction of consonants and vowels, the intonation, the inflection, and rhythmic flow were remarkable. At that moment, *she was her father!* Her copying was

---

1   Daniel N. Stern, *The Interpersonal World of the Infant* (1985), New York: Basic Books.

an un-self-conscious act of love! When her parents laughed with delight at her repeated imitation, she said, "No laugh." How unusual, I thought, for her to say, "No laugh." Is she telling them, "My imitation is not entertainment; it has another meaning"?

I suspect that as she gets older she will think of what she was doing as imitation. She'll adopt her parents' point of view and will have no memory that her imitation was an expression of love. My hope is that at some point in adulthood, she might realize that the underlying feeling of her imitation was love. "Imitation is the sincerest form of flattery" says it well. At her age, imitation was magical! We all learn naturally through this process. Love is, I believe, what feeds the body as a tool. It is not my impression that we think about imitation as love on a conscious level, but the drive to learn through imitation continues unabated through a great part of life, with the anticipation of pleasure. Love as a component of imitation goes mostly unrecognized and/or dismissed. That is why criticism so often hurts. The love is not acknowledged!

Love and the body are intertwined. Love is the essence of movement!

I wonder whether a big part of the emotional pain of physical illness is an unconscious sense that we are losing the body through which we naturally express our love.

— *Imitation and Neurobiology*

In a recent scientific talk at the National Psychological Association for Psychoanalysis by Mary Main,[2] a prominent researcher of attachment theory at the University of California, Berkeley, she mentioned that we register more just by looking at each other in one-twelve-thousandth of a second than we could possibly note on a conscious level.[3] It is hard to imagine that we sense such an incredible amount of information so quickly! And a recent flurry of articles in journals and the popular press concerning the "mirroring neurons"[4] in the brain talk about how imperceptibly our muscles move along with the movements that we are looking at. These brain scan experiments leave little doubt about why this imitative

2   Mary Main. ATWS, the attachment theory website, http://lifecyclejourneys. com/Researchers/MaryMain.

3   http://www.huffingtonpost.com/judith-acosta/lisw-cht/ verbal-first-aid-healing, July 31, 2010.

4   V.S. Ramachandran, "Mirror Neurons and Imitation Learning as the Driving Force Behind 'the Great Leap Forward' in Human Evolution," http://www. edge.org/3rd_culture/ramachandran.

approach is universal. These brain functions evidence a powerful neurobiological component for empathy and serve as the basis for the complex and more conscious development of relatedness as we mature. This is very much a part of what feeds our thinking of the body as a tool.

— *Most Physical Training*

Most training follows a standard format: *do this until you get it right.* Getting it "right" varies with the teacher's orthodoxy, spirit, and sensitivity—from doing it exactly as the teacher does it, to sensing it as it was intended to be or sensing what it was meant to evoke.

Imitation, repetition, repetition, and more repetition are practiced with the expectation that in time the skills will fall into place. Isn't this the way most of us operate? We don't exactly feel what we are doing, yet we unequivocally believe that if we keep doing it our bodies will get it. *Why do we expect our bodies to do what we wish?* As a consequence, we memorize the gestures, the shapes, the sequence, the rhythm, and the emotions of what we are supposed to feel. The *memory of form* becomes a way to repeat. Form is the standard for judging right from wrong! Form is the usual way of talking about the "right" flow of motion: *the hips should be here when the golf club comes up; the elbow should be parallel with the line on the court; the eyes should be looking up and to the right in this position.* The muscles are expected to conform to whatever idea or intention we have in mind!

It is all imitation and repetition and hope!

— *Touching*

In the silent world of dance, as in most physical training, *touching* to adjust the placement of a part of the body is more widespread than explaining. The teaching assumption about the value of touching is, I believe, as follows: touch feeds *body memory.* We have all been held and touched during our infancy to one extent or another. The caretaker's touch gets imprinted in the muscle cells, impacting on our predilection for a particular pressure of touch. I think that we can all attest to this idea of predilection. Some people like a firmer pressure; others, a softer touch. My experience has led me to conjecture that those early imprints determine to a large extent our preferred muscular tonus, tighter or looser muscles, and the activities we gravitate toward.

Imitation and touching build body image and the visualization of internal sensing, both of which construct and reinforce memory. Touch feeds body memory in each of us, tapping into the early infant level of absorption that I addressed earlier.

— Review

Using the body as a tool is thinking of it as the physical way to fulfill a wished-for idea. The body as a tool is supposed to work as an extension of our mind's intention. The body as a tool is indistinguishable from control and memory! Consequently, the awareness of the motion through the muscles, the medium through which actions happen, is seldom, if ever, considered—except for how they can do what we want: *Do I need to make them more flexible or stronger?* We relate to flexibility or strength in terms of what we intend, when we think of the body as a tool.

THE BODY AS AN ORGANISM

— Something Inside

When the body is experienced as an organism, it is thought about as having a life of its own! There is a perpetual monitoring of physiologic sensation: the breath quickening or stopping; the heart pounding; the stomach rumbling. The mind is doing what has evolved into an autonomic system. Something has caused the "body as an organism" person to pay close attention to bodily functions that for the rest of us show up either when we are ill or extremely anxious.

These people are in a persistent state of anxiety, which they have gotten so used to that it is totally normal to them.

— Physical Tendencies

These individuals act with an odd combination of confusion and determination! The lift of the arm while exercising becomes pulling, pulling beyond the point in the body that isn't stretching—the point of resistance. They don't think of the point of resistance as muscle endings. They are intent on overcoming how their body is holding them back from what they think is the purpose of the exercise, namely, going as far into space as one can imagine! The actual sense of elasticity of the muscles, as well as the torques and adjustments to sustain the elastic relationship between muscles in the lift of the arm, is explanatory—but beside the point in the way they are determined to engage their bodies. How far into space one can reach becomes more meaningful than the actual sensation of the musculature. Their psychological wish is freedom to go beyond the body they experience. It became clear to me, through repeated observations, that their reaching out was intent on overcoming some internal physiologic or psychological containment. This type of person experiences his or her body as something that holds the spirit back!

— Assumptions

Early on as a teacher I was always looking to see how my exercise instruction was being assimilated, how closely the students were doing what I thought I had explained and what I was sure I had shown clearly. The "body as organism" students invariably overpulled and overtightend, trying to fulfill, what they were sure, was the ultimate potential of the movement I had shown. The fantasy of the end goal overrode the actuality of what was sensed.

Working hard for flexibility or strength was not uncommon for the vast majority of students in an effort to demand as much of their bodies as possible. But pulling into space as far as they could was especially noticeable with the organism-minded persons.

— Relationship to Me

They were dedicated students who listened with rapt attention, as if I were an elixir to the containment of their demanding organs. The avidness of their interest tended to seduce me by making me feel special. But it became apparent that they were not sensing the specifics of the muscles that I was trying to make clear. They had implicit hope that their intimate sense of me would magically transform them. Most of us could easily relate to this childlike magical expectation, which, in my experience, continued for a long time for the organism person.

— The Fantasy of Motion

For all of the attention paid to physiologic sensations, the relationship to the body is totally mental. Moving out, the sense of motion dominates this type of person's relationship to the body. The *fantasy of motion*—the wish for lightness, the melodic, lyric component of the music—drives their improvisations. The wish for freedom, liberation, for "letting go," is obviously more important than sensing the muscles through which physical motion happens. They do not naturally distinguish their psychological imperatives from the actual muscular sensations of the movements. Physicality and imagination are coupled like an indissoluble chemical compound. Talking about the actual sensation of the muscles is experienced as a dismissal of their primal wish to get away!

The wish for flight is a reversal of the inner containment, of the hidden terror.

✦ A Case in Point ✦

Early on in my curricular creative movement explorations, I encouraged a class of adults to move with the sense of sheer physical weight as they improvised. I did this out of desperation, in an effort to get them to sense their physical selves with greater specificity. Weight, with its heaviness, makes one aware of the sheer physical mass of the body. One student, who moved with the lightness of a willow branch, wound up on the floor after improvising. She rose, voice pitched high with anger. "Why are we doing this?" she asked. "Do you want us to die? This is completely contrary to the feeling of dance."

I was shocked by her reaction to my exploratory effort. I had no idea that I was being so callous! She was assigning a malicious intent to my suggestion to explore weight. She was convinced that it was my unconscious wish to have her experience death. Her experience of weight was a surrender of her emotional survival through airiness! The fear she felt was instantaneously repressed, as she raged, accusing me of wanting her to consciously experience the unthinkable.

Her imagination and judgment were stronger than her actual physical experience. Her thoughts and sensations were entwined like the snakes around Hermes's staff (which, by the way, was a symbol of peace!). The peace that this person was protecting, I later discovered, was an avoidance of the sadness of loss of her father, who had died when she was just twelve years old. It wasn't her feeling of loss, but what I was doing to her that justified her anger. Something had happened to her emotionally that compelled her out-of-control outburst! She was surprised by the fear she expressed. Paradoxically, this particular student had always thought of me as a fantastic movement teacher!

— Muscles and Fear

Her emotional avoidance of fear pulled her skeletal muscles inward, lifting the spine like a ballet dancer, a skeletal component of my earlier reference to the willow-branch lightness of her movement. Her experience with weight momentarily broke through her physically patterned, unconscious personality defense.

— An Empty Space

The tightness of the muscles creates an empty-space body—an imagined floating space of organs between the bones and the skin! Although this sort of person moves lightly, they think of themselves as heavy. They are usually flexible because, as I mentioned, they are persistently pulling away from the spine and joints, experiencing the mass or texture of the musculature as undifferentiated from body hinges. In the exercises, they are particularly responsive to spatial directives, such as, "Turn the palm of the right arm up as you stretch with your left arm to the left side," which they easily visualize as they pull into the direction of the gesture as if the direction into space is the feeling of the exercise, as if their imagined intention is the feeling.

— The Imaginative Mind

Paradoxically, on the upside of this empty but heavy body is an imagined lightness that derives from the way these people relate to energy—like moths to the light! The way their minds have come to work overshadows the mass of their bodies. Heavy and light are determined by the mind vacillating between being carried by the energy of imagined associations or descending into an unmanageable organism.

The sense of motion, the flow of motion, is what speaks to them, in contrast to the "body as a tool" person for whom the defining experience of movement is the concrete boundaries of form. Inherent in the sense of motion is an empty space, opening without constraints to receive their embracing gestures.

— Imagined Space

The student who was denying the loss of her father never truly separated, as if death were not the end! She maintained a wished-for, idealized father, an idealization that fed her airiness, her emotional defense against sadness and the anger of loss. Space unites! These individuals relate to me more than to their own bodies, not unlike an infant gazing at the mother. They are aesthetically appreciative yet lack a definitive personal opinion, as they *talk* about what they are connecting to, rather than connecting to their own feelings.

Once again, the mind subordinates the actuality of the muscular experience of movement. Imagination trumps reality!

— *The Process that Transforms*
The first separation in the Genesis story of creation is heaven from earth. Making the organism person aware of the feet's contact to the floor helps them in a very concrete way to experience the body from the floor up, in contrast to their usual imaginative way of experiencing the body from the top down. This process slowly impacts on the interplay of muscles, leading to their ability to distinguish motion from emotion.

Because the ground is such a "now" sensation, the imaginative mind of these people, which had helped to control their experience of terror by enabling them to escape into the openness of space, now helps them to feel a physical solidity that can withstand whatever it was that was so scary in their childhood.

THE BODY AS A CHANNEL

— *Energy Driven*
The person who experiences the body as a channel believes that his or her muscular sensations are urges, signals registering in the body. These urges vary from impulses coming from within the body to sensory vibes coming from outside. The body is an antenna receiving signals! The impulse signals are what most people call a gut feeling, an under-the-skin sensation that takes over, overshadowing the wholeness of the body. You can think of it as places in the body that become focal points of energy generating power of their own, not unlike a Hindu *chakra*. The sensory vibrations are like impulses that the person has a sense of coming from the outside rather than from inside the body. These messages, whether coming from the unconscious or some other intangible place, demand acknowledgement and release. The messages feel urgent, bordering on compulsions to act or react! The stronger the urge, the more tenuous is the control of the sensed energy.

There is no question in the "channel body" mind that he/she is totally in their body.

✦ *A Case in Point* ✦

An accomplished movement-skilled student would almost invariably mop her face with the palm of her hand at some point in her improvisation or thrust her palm outward to ward off an imaginary force. The gestures always had the urgent force of an internal impulse. She thought it was anger. But at some point I thought that her effort to remove her facial features, might be fear. She was stunningly beautiful, but behaved as if this was insignificant, as if her beauty or regard for her good looks got in the way of the seriousness of ideas and what she truly felt. She heard the music quite accurately, but her improvisation was driven by energy from inside demanding expulsion! It was the exploration of impulses underneath or within a gesture and the exploration of centers—focal areas within the torso—that most intrigued her.

The musculature for the channel person vibrates. And just as space is of the essence for the organism person, *time* is what dictates the improvisations of the channel person. It is not time in the ordinary beat/rhythm organization of sound, but condensed time, compressed time. Their movement takes on a pressured effort, vacillating between contained and forceful gestures, as they wait for the emanation of new energies. They do not sense disconnects in their body because the internal forces give them a sense of a togetherness, as if their bodies are glued together by forces that can be guided but not controlled. Of course, they say, "I feel my muscles!" They visualize a tension in the musculature, like the wiring armature of a clay sculpture.

— *Separate, yet Physically Locked In*

I have hypothesized that the channel person has, in growing up, made a connection between their reaction to something coming from the outside that they resisted and a parallel internal, physical sensation that they registered as a signal. The context that generated the physical signal is forgotten, but the signal that alerts the fight-or-flight response remains. They think of themselves as unquestionably separate, independent, almost to a fault. I have corroborated this hypothesis over the years, as some of them have shared their history with me. Their impulses serve to protect them from the power of others whose energies or influences need to be deflected, so as not to be killed, swallowed, or from something harmful that needs to be warded off! However, their physicality suggests a persistent guardedness that locks them into an attachment that has no name.

The sense of such enormous power extended to someone or something is by its nature very childlike. There is a paranoiac flavor to these channel persons. But make no mistake; these experiences are as real to them as the pain of hunger for an infant, which always manifests as urgent. The physiology of infantile hunger is the base template for compulsions, as well as intuitions, that are experienced as equally instant!

— *Impulses and Identity*

I, the teacher, am understood as an external energy field, as if I were speaking in code. Impulses speak through me, just as impulses speak through them. Nothing is what it seems like on the surface! The outside, the external, is but a faint expression of the inner world. They never exactly follow instructions—and almost invariably justify their divergence as something their body needs to do.

— *A Way of Thinking*

Back in the late sixties at an end-of-the-year school concert, I spoke about my exploration of space through the exploration of centers in the body. Centers are a simple enough notion that has the dancer visualize an area within the head and/or torso from which connective lines emanate throughout the body. The visualization of each center has the effect of evoking a different sense of space, in contrast to the traditional visual, directional division of space. I had begun to explore this sort of creative spatial experience with the fourteen and fifteen-year-olds. The mother of a younger child, who was in the audience, approached me after the concert and asked how I had arrived at the notion of centers. I described my personal experience in a matter-of-fact way, after which she insisted that I was one of the chosen few human beings through whom certain universal truths were revealed! From her perspective, tuning in to the body is a language of universal forces, and I was one of the chosen messengers through whom this knowledge was to be disseminated. From her perspective, I was endowed with a channel body.

— *An Ancient Tradition*

The awareness of the body giving us physiological signals is not only true in medical science, but derives from an ancient tradition of believing that forces in the universe pass through the body. Psychosomatics, a psychological understanding of physical symptoms that express repressed emotional conflicts, is in keeping with this ancient tradition. These traditions treat the musculature physiologically as disease, kinesiologically as muscles moving bones, or psychologically as evoking an infantile kinesthesia. The interplay of muscles—the conscious connectedness that realigns the musculature and can be consciously developed—is totally unknown.

Both memory and control drive the central experience of the self, the body self, for the channel person.

— *The Stabilizing Force*

Contact of the feet with the floor is a profound stabilizing force. The weight of the body gives substance to the contact with the earth. The equation of contact supporting weight becomes the anchor for the channel mind, which makes assumptions about physical signals. The contact is like connecting the flowering mind to its root by adding a stem! Another stabilizing factor is the awareness of the breath that serves to mitigate the pressure that the channel person applies to the feet's contact with the floor. Both breath and contact are the dominant factors that bring the channel person to the awareness of the interplay of muscles.

✦ Case in Point ✦

I am reminded of an impressively sensitive student moving around in a large studio, on a hot summer day, with an open forty-eight-inch window on the tenth floor. Back in the eighties, I was not as clear about what I now have the words to describe, but I sensed this particular woman functioning from this unknown otherworldly place. I walked over to the window unobtrusively to lower it for fear that she might just throw herself out, without realizing it, as if sleep walking. This student had been duly honored and rewarded for her incredible sensibilities and scholarship. She once told me that faced with an emotionally frightening situation that made her feel as though she would go crazy, she repeated my emphasis on keeping foot contact with the floor like a mantra, and it saved her from going mad! She was factually dealing with a life-threatening attachment to someone she loved very deeply. Loss was an unbearable thought.

It made me realize how profound contact with the floor is beyond my own concrete, seemingly prosaic use of this suggestion as an initial approach to help students differentiate the elasticity of muscles to facilitate the eventual interplay of muscles.

— From Psychic Sensibility to Tactile Perception

Once again I want to make clear that these individuals relate to the body from a mind-driven frame of reference. They are seemingly not denying the body, but are not attuned to the specificity of the musculature. The contracted, misaligned musculature is treated metaphorically as a center or as a message. They create a meaning that dictates the physical experience. The body is turned into a mythic temple—the term Martha Graham used to refer to the body. The musculature for the channel person is a vibration rather than a tactile, tangible reality.

— The Transformative Process

It is exactly this distinction that makes contact of the feet with the floor so important in helping to differentiate between the imagined and the actual, between suspicion and feeling, between believing that one is beyond a shadow of a doubt separate and being personal.

THE POSSESSIVE MIND

The most difficult subjects can be explained to the most slow-witted man if he has not formed any idea of them already; but the simplest thing cannot be made clear to the most intelligent man if he is firmly persuaded that he knows already, without a show of doubt, what is laid before him.

Leo Tolstoy

THE SUBORDINATION OF THE BODY

I use the above quote because I am asking you to consider ways of thinking and functioning that all of us grow up with, treat as our nature, and never question!

After a significant breakthrough a few years ago, a student of mine, whose arthritic condition and underlying terror altered dramatically, sent this unsolicited quote to me. She asked, "Why doesn't everyone teach this way?"

It seems like a perfectly reasonable question to ask, since the interplay of muscles transformed her way of sensing and thinking about motion and how it touched her emotionally.

It took me close to thirty years to grasp and refine teaching this way. This started in 1959, when Jeffrey, the seven-year-old referred to in the opening page of this book, did his dance improvisation of "clay," which led to *Creative Movement for Children: A Dance Program for the Classroom,* published in 1969, and which spearheaded the opening of the School for Creative Movement (1962-1992) and continues in small private classes to this day. Those forty-one explorative and inventive years produced a creative-movement syllabus that covered students from preschoolers to adults enrolled in a seven-year graduate program. It also included my certification as a psychoanalyst after an eleven-year training program. The psychoanalytic literature reveals what we have come to know and practice to facilitate getting in touch with parts of ourselves that we may not have thought about and with how those parts feed into our daily lives. This combination of creative movement and psychoanalysis led to understanding how to get people to not only feel uninhibited while moving but more significantly experience the improvisation emotionally.

ATTACHMENT-MEMORY-CONTROL

I have come to understand three fundamental ways of thinking that stand out as to why we don't pay attention to the interplay of muscles as a natural, given gateway for the emanation of feelings. The first is *attachment,* a profound, emotionally laden process for survival and learning of trust, that continues to be used physically, albeit unconsciously, beyond the point where it is helpful.

— *A Typical Response*
You can easily see attachment in the way someone begins to move to a piece of music, settling into the phrasing, moving on certain beats, while holding other beats, or sensing accents or downbeats, to repeat over and over again. Phrasing feels safe! The body and the music feel comfortably related. This very common relationship is an expression of attachment. It is how most people dance to music.

— *A Need for Closeness*
For some, the phrasing is not enough. They have an emotional pull to get closer to the more complicated inner rhythms or their imagined spatial sense of the music. One can see this stronger connection with older teenagers and young adults for whom finding connection is a big part of their lives. Think of the premise and success of Facebook.

Dance students have this compelling relationship to attachment that elevates imitation to an aesthetic ideal in the profession. The professional dancer works very hard to make the attachment personal, artful, and emotionally safe. Doing so requires a high degree of flexibility and the ability to control muscles quickly. The dancer is trained in memory and control, which are the other two fundamental natural functions that we don't question in relationship to the body.

— *The Nonphysical Attachment*

Connecting to the musical phrasing is a minimal physical adjustment. There are lots of people who do not want to adjust muscularly! We have all felt that lack of desire to adjust when we were very angry or disappointed or deeply saddened, all of which made us cold and distant. When these emotions are successfully repressed and controlled, at all cost, there is no wish to dance. Movement is subsequently reduced to actions that are goal oriented, like tennis, golf, or ballroom dancing. These activities are fundamentally committed to mastery and control. We judge the cleanliness of form, the coolness of demeanor. The attachment to these activities may be passionate, but the emotional experience of the motion is invariably judged in terms of what is wished for, not what is felt.

Control becomes a prized character trait!

— *Dancing Is a Choice*

Most dancing requires adjusting to the music, to a partner, to an imagined fantasy. A lot of people do not move, and rationalize it as a choice, which explains why a lot of people have spinal tension that shows up psychosomatically in millions of new visits to chiropractors yearly for back pain![5] In 2006 musculoskeletal symptoms were the number-two reason for physicians visits.[6]

DANCING ATTACHMENTS

— *Tempo*

Attaching to the tempo, the spirit of the music is easier from a muscular perspective. Relating to the imagined sense of a piece of music registers mostly in movements of the head and neck, arms and torso, characterized by swaying "sections" of the body: the head–neck, the rib cage–arms, hip–torso, while the legs remain more or less stationary. It is flowing, romantic, moving to one's fantasy of the music, the imagined space of the music, moving in the way the music is telling them to move!

---

5   ACA, "Facts About Chiropractic, Back Pain, Facts and Statistics," http://acatoday.org/press.

6   AAOS, "Your Orthopedic Connection," http://orthoinfo.aaos.oorg/topic.cfm, May 2009.

✦ A Case in Point ✦

A music-loving student would for many years react to my observations about her connection of muscles as a contradiction to what the music is saying. She loved music and felt certain that her response was exactly what the music wanted of her. I learned at some point that she sensed without questioning exactly what her parents wanted of her! This unquestioned sense of certainty about what is wanted informed her professionally to become a very respected voice in child psychiatry.

The goal of the tempo-attachment person in exercising is flexibility; the dance goal is freedom through space, like the famous Isadora Duncan wrapped in flowing diaphanous fabric, floating around the stage.

The conviction of certainty about the music is psychological not actual. Music can be interpreted in many different ways. The tempo person treats the music like someone who is asking or demanding something from them, which they must try to fulfill.

Psychotherapists often wonder what the patient unconsciously wants from them, as if they are the wished-for parent (this is called *transference*), or what they want from the patient (referred to as the *counter-transference*).

— Rhythms

Rhythms, the inner play on the beat of the music, are more demanding of the musculature and nervous system. Rhythms involve the speed of tightening and loosening muscles. The feet and legs are the main movers. Latin music, usually rhythmic, is mostly danced to with feet and hip movements. The upper torso moves but is contained. MTV dancing, which is rhythm driven, is characterized by quick releases and containment of sections of the body reassembled into split-second frozen shapes. Think of Michael Jackson unleashing motion and strikingly containing it.

Rhythmic attachment is closer to ritual tribal dancing in which the drums are dictating the speed of the spirit. The musculature is "sacrificed" to a collective impulse, not unlike the Woodstock Music Festival in 1969, where the mass of people and music became a whirlpool of intoxication; or the roar of the crowd at a football game; or the more mild enthusiasm of a parade. The rhythmic attachment is primitive and stamped with urgency, like an infant's reaction to a disturbing stimulus. It is an unconscious time warp!

Let me explain. Both tempo and rhythm attachments are profoundly psychological. The body is automatically given over to the organization of the music, like children who give themselves over to the parental emotional tempo and rhythm, which they come to enjoy as they learn to handle these emotional states. This automatic psychophysical attachment happens most profoundly under the age of two.

The parent to whom these attachments were made are usually forgotten; what remains are personality predispositions on a sensory level to the tempo or rhythm or, ironically, to the repressed conflict expressed in the unwillingness to dance.

Both tempo and rhythm attachments are characterized by anxiety. Connections are and need to be made quickly. The muscles are not considered. The physical self is subsumed by the patterned character response. The unconscious fantasy is omniscience, knowing what is wanted and needs to be done.

✦ *A Case in Point* ✦

A thirtysomething moves stunningly like a shark in water, muscles in constant motion. She couldn't distinguish the speed of motion from the awareness of the interplay of muscles.

A fiftysomething with a background in dance invariably spins to the timing of the music. She has a talent for attunement to others. She finds the awareness of the interplay inhibiting to her freedom, as if the body should accompany her desired attitude about dance.

THE LOSS OF SELF

These natural patterns of attachment to the music are so common that no one sees that there is an implicit lack of self-awareness. *The relationship—the attachment—becomes the focus.* The irrefutable self in movement—the musculature—is unconsciously split off, in the service of the relationship. The musculature is used, *has to be used,* but there is no conscious sensitivity of the motion moving through muscles, from muscle to muscle, as they engage the relationship to the music. The sensitivity to muscles is subsumed by the focus on the sensory experience or the interpreted meaning of it, which are judgments about movement.

— Patterns

People use patterns of movement with no sense of whether the motion is or is not moving through the lower back or the pelvis or whatever part of the body is disconnected, partially engaged, or engaged sometimes and not at other times. Whenever some sections of the body are used and not others, the clarity of feelings moving naturally through the muscles is split off. Physical patterned habits are entrenched emotional disconnects. They are the reason for physical aches, pains, and eventual medical interventions that demand that someone do something to them—for them!

— Rationalizations

When the body doesn't make the relationship to the music easily, judgments are turned against the self: *"I started dancing too late," "I'm too stiff," "I wish I could but I am socially inhibited,"* or the rejecting denial, *"I don't like to dance."* We tend to accept these rationalizations because there is some modicum of truth about them. These rationalizations are telling expressions of conflicts that have not been dealt with and which show up in misaligned musculature: *"I will not look at why I can't focus on my muscles, even though I know that they are what I use to move." "I would rather continue to experience a disjointed, dissociated physical self than deal with the attachment conflicts my body safeguards."*

These rationalizations further evidence the misplaced/displaced body, the dismissal of misalignments that could be worked with and that involve a separation from the attachment body.

— The Denial

It is not the feelings of the music that people usually relate to—but how the music is organized. It parallels listening to words without sensing the feelings that the words are being used to express. The primacy of the muscular experience is overshadowed by the mind registering sensations, choices, and meaning.

Muscular contractions as the primal psychophysical defense against feelings are what reign supreme.

NATURAL DEVELOPMENTS

Control and memory are natural developments of the mind that also subordinate the awareness of feelings flowing through the interplay of muscles. Control and memory are invaluable for our maturity. They are both highly prized, personally and culturally.

— *Memory and Body*

The repetition of sensations is what develops as body memory. Repeatedly sucking at the breast or the nipple of a bottle is what allows the infant to use the movement of the cheeks and tongue to imagine sucking at the breast to stave off hunger. Anyone who has witnessed an infant reflexively using his or her facial muscles and tongue just prior to crying with hunger will attest to what I am noting. A day-old newborn can turn its head to respond to the direction of a sound,[7] away from the breast, suggesting, as was pointed out when I listened to details on this experiment, that we are born with a somatosensory system hardwired for independence.

The senses and muscles work together from the very beginning of life.

The repetition of these sensory/muscular experiences becomes the template for body memory. The subsequent ability to split the muscles from the senses becomes control. The lips and tongue can become dissociated from hunger and associated with the person who gratifies the hunger. Using the lips and tongue as a means for pleasure, a memory of muscles; turning the head can be dissociated from responding to the direction of a stimulus and becomes an expression of shame or an insistent "no," once again, *a memory to be mastered and controlled*. Muscles dissociated, isolated from the wholeness of their original functions, become memory for control.

Looked at from this perspective, both memory and control are unavoidable aspects of our learning process. The control of the muscles allows us to disconnect from the original processes and objects in which they came into play and instead to use them to express a variety of intentions. This unconscious disconnect process establishes a bodily sense of self or a "body ego,"[8] as Freud described. And this in turn helps us to develop a boundary between self and others.

Individuality becomes unwittingly bound to muscular resistance!

---

7   Ibid. Mary Main.
8   Sigmund Freud, *The Ego and the Id* (1923), W. W. Norton & Company.

The muscular, resistant self-pattern, defined by control and memory, continues to function unconsciously in relationship to other objects, our fantasies, and ideas.

Memory and control are the Siamese twins of liberation from dependency, in charge of distinguishing pleasure from pain, self from other, and attitudes from emotions. What is not realized in this self-isolating process is that our inborn, natural muscular empathy is diminished

The pride in this isolation, which disparages the awareness of wholeness, never quite extinguishes the early kinesthetic experience. The natural wholeness is displaced in the togetherness of mass events: rock concerts, the wave at a football game; or elevated into notions of Nirvana, the Garden of Eden. The feelings traveling through the muscles are subordinated to sensations, memory, and control that feed the intellectual mind.

We collect and classify memory, creating folders of experience. *Memory is a way to control.* It is central to education. It is central to expectations. Memory functions to make the infant feel safe. Memory is the past being used in the present for security.

A question for the reader: *Do we fear losing our memory—or the control that memory gives us the illusion of having?*

Controlling sensation becomes an unwitting repression of feelings. Remembering sensation becomes an unwitting substitute for feeling!

BODY MEMORY

Most of us depend on our musculature to respond automatically to our intentions. The learning curve between nerves, muscles, and brain happens so early in life that we are mostly unconscious of it and it is usually forgotten. It is replaced by an overarching sense we call body memory, treated as akin to a reflex—which it is not, though it feels that way. Practically everyone moves from the perspective of body memory: stepping on the beat, swaying to the melody, shifting from side to side to the phrasing of the music. The muscles are expected to follow.

Body memory is what feeds *imaging* the body! We compose a picture of the body in our mind. We image front, back, inside, outside, and so on. Some people retain the connection between memory and sensation. They *visualize* the image of the front of the body, the connection between head and fingers. Memory fires the nerves, producing a sensation that makes the memory feel alive!

Body memory for a baseball pitcher is visualizing his arm and leg wind up into the release of the ball; it is a sequence of motion. Retraining a pitcher's delivery is not easy because the motion develops into an instinctual delivery that feels like a reflex. Getting pitchers to sense even a slight shift in the way their pitching arms come up takes an incredible amount of practice, as any coach will swear. The more attuned the person is to sensations, the easier the retraining, because they can more easily sense the subtlety of the shift in the motion of the muscles.

✦ A Case in Point ✦

I once had a rather disturbed patient who refused to talk about the past because recalling felt the same to him as experiencing the moment. For him memory and sensation felt inextricably connected, like a vine clinging to a tree trunk. The psychological work with him was extremely practical.

During a dance workshop a young woman reacted to sensing the weight of her body by telling me, "I feel the earth is pulling me down!"

In both of these cases, sensation is tied into a memory expressing an ongoing struggle with separation from an internal attachment, one so powerful that the need for control is paramount to survival. There was no sense for these individuals of being present in their bodies. Body memory enveloped their experience.

— Imaging and Visualization

Imaging and visualization are dependent on the memory of a constructed body map. The body map is drawn by visually placing sensations on body parts: front, back, side, diagonal, top, bottom, in, out; and sensations of time: fast and slow; and temperature: hot and cold, giving volume to *form*, the sine qua non of professional dance and the abstractions of scholarship.

— Form

Form is a body map. The map may be connected through the sensory activation of visualization or imaging physical volume. Form is an aesthetic standard in all body-based disciplines: dance, yoga, tai chi, and so on. Form is what is traditionally taught as the gateway to the wisdom under the surface of memory and sensation! When the sensations connected to memory are demonstrated in the form, the student is considered talented. Because feelings are recalled as sensations (the assumption of metaphors!), it sometimes happens that feelings *do* come through the sensations, resulting in artistry! Those moments—those events—are transcendent, and one has to be ready to receive them!

The irony is that neither form nor sensations equal feeling. *Feelings do not have form*. Form is the end product of the organic flow of feelings. Forms are remembrances for the sake of control. Form exists in imagination and for the sake of authority!

— *Form and Directions*

If you follow my thinking of how experience becomes intellectual, conceptual, and metaphorical, you can understand why movement is then thought of in terms of form and direction. Intentions are associated with direction: *"You can tell she's ashamed by the way she is 'pulling away"* or *"I am determined to go forward."* We look and assess movement in terms of space and time, a trajectory that has intention and therefore meaning. The fact that *movement happens through the muscles*, through the interplay of muscles, is unwittingly or arrogantly treated as insignificant to the meaning that the self or the viewer assigns to the gestures or the tension of form. The musculature through which feelings are expressed is usually not even seen, although I fully believe it is subliminally sensed, despite the intellectual dominance of immediately reducing gesture into symbolic meaning.

Meaning is too often a form of distancing self from feelings.

— *Forms and Gestures*

Imaging and visualizations are the groundswells of imagination: for the Spaniard Pablo Picasso, it was a nose on the side of a face to accentuate its prominence both as a visual actuality and as a metaphor about the person; for the Dutch painter Piet Mondrian it was colored rectangles and squares to represent the streets of New York, replicating his familiarity with the geometry of Holland's landscape; and for the American poet E. E. Cummings, it was eliminating punctuation to convey a process of mind that was not logical and linear, not declarative, but more like dissociated dream images.

These forms, these aesthetic gestures, are a language to express feelings that the artist has about his subject. If the forms and gestures truly convey the feelings, the work becomes transcendent, and the forms and gestures disappear; if they dominate, then the craft, the concept, the abstraction has successfully obscured the feelings. We—the viewers, the readers, the listeners—may be impressed, appreciative, or critical, but we miss the human communication.

— Abstract Thinking

Even abstract thinking depends on body memory for its vitality. The word *hope* is an abstraction! Hope is an expectation that things will turn out well. Hope is based on the memories of living through and surviving. When the feelings of pain and terror are overwhelming rather than the expectation of survival, then abstractions, like hope, feel empty. There are many people for whom hope does not spring eternal. Abused children, as an example, have no memory of comfort—and consequently have no hope. It is very difficult to foster hope in such people.

Abstractions condense the memory of experience. When abstractions are used without illustrative examples there is an expectation that the listener will fill in the missing pieces.

EXPECTATIONS

The mother's empathic response to the crying child is based on the body memory of her own pain. What fuels the usual frustrating anger between husbands and wives are expectations of the other's empathy. The unacknowledged expectation of another's body memory is how infants and toddlers behave. When abstractions are used without verbalizing the feelings that support them, they betray a childlike expectation by the person using them. It is this understanding of the unspoken expectations that serves therapists in their work.

— Thinking Without Feeling

When there is an expectation that the body will follow easily from a thought, it is fair to say that cognition, or thought, trumps the sensory process of the body. Or to put it psychologically, fantasy trumps the actuality of feeling. Fantasy is an imaginative extension of body memory. Getting at feelings through ideas is no simple matter; and this is why art therapies become so useful as an intermediary process toward consciousness. Art therapies elicit the unverbalized experience in a way that talking therapies require more interaction to make resonant.

— Cognition and Fantasy

Both cognition and fantasy often distort perception. The distortion is the belief, as with my disturbed patient who refused to talk about the past, that the sensory memory of an experience is the same as feelings. Instead of being alive to the feelings in the experience of remembering, they are alive to the recollected judgment about the sensation. *But remembering feeling is not the same as feeling.*

— In Movement

Memory narrows the experience of movement. Memory is not the thing itself! Using muscle memory is external, the choreography, like the written play. It is the aliveness to feelings that makes the play or the choreography come alive. Warming up facilitates the sensibility to the musculature through which feelings travel.

If the interplay of muscles does not come into play in movement, then the feelings do not emanate into our awareness. Feelings are there because they function like circulation—but their light is dimmed.

THE PARADOX

Ironically, according to the latest brain research,[9] memory is constantly being put together in the moment; and that is why memory is never quite the same! We have all experienced lapses of memory—most especially when strong emotions are rattling something inside of us below the surface of whatever is going on.

So much depends on what is going on under the surface. Feelings are why awareness is so important and useful. Awareness or sensitivity to the musculature, especially the interplay of muscles, is what my fifty-year experience with movement has shown me is the generator of creativity and a resolution for the rigidity of memory.

The rigidity of memory is apparent when someone gets stuck dancing to the beat of music because they are relating to the musical

---

9   Antonio Damasio, *The Feeling of What Happens: Body and Emotion in the Making of Consciousness* (1999), Harvest/Harcourt, Inc.

organization and not to their own feeling or even the feeling of the music.

The notation of the beats, the organization of the music, is a way to capture the feelings, a way to remember. It is not the feeling! In jazz, improvising on the beat is to express the feeling with the memory of the music. Conductors of symphonies do the same with the coloration and textures of sound. This is the essence of their individuality, of their insight into the feeling of a piece of music.

When you walk without the awareness of the ground coming up through your muscles, you are not alive to your feelings. Your body is treated as an addendum to your intentions or that part of you that holds your spirit back.

Technique, remembering, will never substitute for the spontaneous, artfulness of feeling.

WITH THE MUSCLES

The mind is not, in and of itself, possessive. It is obviously a gift of nature. But when attachment, memory, and control dominate our sensory/muscular self, the split becomes a detriment to the constancy of our feeling awareness, the light of the enlightened self.

FOR EVERYONE, EVERYWHERE THE INTERPLAY OF MUSCLES

What follows is my specific approach to integrating the fourth-toe-line contact into an incremental realignment of the musculature throughout the body. Slowly and carefully do what you are about to read. Do not rush through this process. You are making changes that are transformative physically and, as you will experience with repeated practice, emotionally.

THE INITIAL FIFTEEN EXERCISES

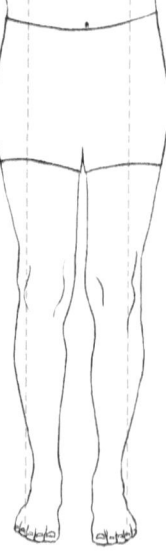

1. **Start by standing with your feet hips-width apart, over the fourth-toe line of the feet.**
2. **Flex your knees slightly and blow out through your mouth several times until you sense a drop in your torso and neck, a sense of weight falling down through your body.**

   Breathing out is a general release of the tension of the muscles held in the spine, shoulders, and neck. The resulting sense of weight (heaviness) should be maintained throughout all of the subsequent exercises.

   This generalized relaxation of the musculature will allow you to sense the motion of movement in a muscle.

   It is this perception of the motion through a muscle that makes whatever you do truly personal and specific.

Sensing the motion in a muscle will allow you to channel the motion from muscle to muscle and most carefully in the torque around a joint. This is the process of muscular realignment. It is the interplay of muscles.

3. **Go up on your toes a very tiny bit (called a *demi-releves*) several times. You will quickly note if one of your ankles stiffens faster than the other, which means that the motion, the alignment, through that foot and ankle is insecure.**
Realigning the forty muscles and twenty-seven bones in each foot so that your arch remains truly strong and supportive of standing over the fourth-toe line takes sensitivity. Your patience will be amply rewarded as feet and ankle strains disappear.

4. **Move the leg of your weaker ankle in closer to your other leg, narrowing your stance.**
Do this incrementally until rising up on your toes no longer stiffens either ankle.

Don't be surprised if, at the beginning of making these small adjustments, you have to do demi-releves many, many times before getting a clear sense of the symmetry of sensation in both ankles.

Your perception of the motion through the muscles of your feet and ankles is constantly changing and needs to be reestablished anew each time. It is this awareness of establishing your perception of the motion anew that keeps you in the here and now.

In making the adjustment of how close your legs need to be to each other for the motion of movement to pass smoothly without any stiffening, you are finding the absolutely perfect narrowing of your stance.

This perfect narrowing between your legs assures that your balance is

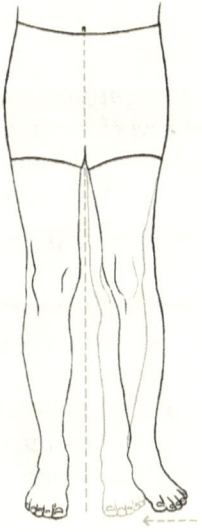

suspended through the interplay of muscles, rather than rigidly held by stiffening joints.

Your brain registers this suspension as the feeling of motion ascending, rather than lifting.

This distinction shifts your consciousness to what you are sensing, along with what you are doing.

5. **It is also likely that one of the toes in one foot will stiffen faster than the other. Swivel those toes in from the heel inward toward the other foot.**
   - Swivel incrementally. Remember that you are asking forty small muscles and twenty-seven bones in the foot to readjust to each other.
   - It may be necessary to swivel inward with the other foot as well.
   - *Do not move the heels* as you swivel your toes.
   - You have now found the just-right placement of your feet and legs that promotes the correct alignment of muscles, registering in the brain that you are grounded and supported.

   Only this clarity facilitates the relaxation of neck, shoulders, and spine muscles that held us up as an infant.
   - *You are shifting from an infantile sense of balance through rigidity to an adult capacity for balance through suspension through the musculature, like a suspension bridge.*

✦ A Case in Point ✦

An eighty-plus-year-old woman with one replaced knee and one, as the MRI showed, on the verge of collapse, has been able for the last ten years to dance and improvise based on learning how to distribute her effort through the interplay of muscles into the suspension, thus avoiding aggravating the collapsing knee.

6. **Staying over the** *whole* **fourth-toe line, bend forward and down with your torso, flexing your knees slightly.**

   - Keep bending your knees so that the point of resistance as you stretch your lower back, buttocks, thighs, and calves is loosened enough to sense the muscles above and below that point.

- By not pulling at a point of resistance, you help to integrate the relationship between muscles, like connecting notes in music. You are facilitating the interplay of muscles.
- Shift your pelvis incrementally left or right, so as to experience the symmetry of sensation between right and left sides, correcting the compensatory misalignments that your body made without your realizing it.
- Your brain automatically shifts muscles throughout the body to balance and avoid falling. This evolutionary system does not care whether it creates peculiar compensations that distort your alignment.
- Our internal evolutionary system is fundamentally dedicated to survival, with very little interest in the wholeness of the expression of feelings. That is why consciousness has always been a choice.
- *Whatever amount of incremental adjustments you make as you work in this way is corrective, cumulative, bringing you closer to the kinesthetic sensibility, to the feeling body.*

It is quite obvious to me as I write out these instructions and commentary, how wordy the process is to make the "natural" conscious. The child in me wishes that there were an easier, magical way to achieve awareness. But the fifty years of experience with the relationship of body and psyche tells me that it just doesn't work that way.

— *Continuing the Exercises*
- Bend over for forty-eight counts to slowly stretch the many muscles involved.
- Come up with your torso, making sure to stay over the fourth-toe line of the feet.
- You'll find that the knees don't quite straighten if you stay over the *whole line* on the soles of your feet.
- Do not press your knees back to straighten, because you unwittingly lock the ankle and knee joints, pushing back onto your heels, stiffening to satisfy the *idea* of straight. Try not to lose the elastic sense in the muscles.
- Straighten by sensing a torque from the muscles of your feet around the outside of your ankles into the outer lower part of the calf muscles.

- Proceed slowly, doing only as much as what you sense. The torque will increase and become clearer with repeated awareness.
- The torque continues around the outside of your knees into the rotation of your thighs and eventually under the buttock into the perineum, in the middle of your pelvis.
- This rotation takes time to develop incrementally.
- Ballet instruction too often forces this process by postural positioning, eventuating in arthritic problems. You do not have to study ballet to have the same arthritic problems occur. Intolerable fear contracts the musculature deeply into the body. *You may continue to function in this same fearful way as an adult by thinking that figuring things out with your mind is all you need to do, never noticing what the muscles are doing.*
- Learn to perceive how much those muscles are capable of rotating in relationship to each other.
- *Perceiving how your muscles connect one to the other is your best defense against following instructions blindly whether they come from the outside or from yourself.*
- If you force the torque and rotation, your knees, hips, and lower back compensate for the weakness in the interplay of muscles.
- Knowing about your trauma and fear will not in itself alter the body's natural defense of contractions to self protect. *You have to deal with nature's process directly for it not to become a second-nature problem.*

2. **Lift your arms up above your shoulders, palms facing each other. Reaching through the fingertips with an emphasis on the back of the hand and the interplay to the top of the forearm, stretch the sides of your torso for a count of eight. Reach over to your side for eight counts, and then to the other side for eight counts, and finally back to the center for eight counts.**
It takes about eight seconds for all of the strands of a muscle to participate in an action. This is why eight is so woven into the organization of Western music.
Repeat the whole sequence: thirty-two down, four up, four right, four left, four up; sixteen down, two, two, two, two; eight down, one, one, one, one; four, one, one, one, one; and

last, two down, one up, one side, one other side, one up; and bend down stretching for eight counts.

This sequence heals lower back problems by facilitating the interplay of muscles between the middle and lower back, under the buttocks, and from the thighs to the feet.

✦ *A Case in Point* ✦

A fiftysomething female student who had been suffering for years with a lordosis (a concave lower back), which she attributed to "that's how I'm built!," found herself exercising without any fear of aggravating her "natural" inheritance.

3. **Keeping your hands flat or your fingertips on the floor, stick your buttocks up in the air to stretch the back of the thighs only as much as you can without stiffening your knees.**
   - This simply changes the point of origin of the stretch.
4. **While still bent over, bring your arms behind your back and clasp your fingers keeping the heels of your hands together.**
   - Pull up and out towards your head.
   - When your shoulders stiffen, bend your knees. This releases the generalized pressure of the stiffening.
   - Pull out again. Bend again; and then pull out one last time.
   - Keeping your arms pulled out, lift your torso up to straighten; making sure to stay over the fourth-toe line, knees will remain slightly flexed.
5. **With your fingers still clasped, bring your arms to your right while turning your head left, and then reverse this position. Do this twice. Release your clasped fingers and let your arms fall to your sides.**
6. **Lift your straight arms out in front just below chest level.**
   - Swing them back to just above shoulder level. Do this eight times.

✦ A Case in Point ✦

A woman in her sixties came back to class, after a hiatus of more than thirty years, with a severe rheumatoid arthritic condition that had already required a shoulder cusp operation. It was impossible for her to follow the above directions. I suggested that she move her arms both in front and to the back only within her comfortable range of motion, using the limitation as a guide, but never losing the interplay of muscles coming from the fourth-toe line. This permission and guidance incorporated into the improvisation sustained her incredible dream of dancing. Three years later, the physical phenomenology of her fear, the profundity of which I am not at liberty to share, is 99 percent gone, as is her muscular rigidity.

7. **Swing the right arm forward and around four times, like a pendulum, and then back and around four times.**
   - Repeat this sequence with your left arm four times
   - Repeat this sequence with both arms four times.
8. **Stretch your arms to the sides slightly below shoulder level. Rotate your fingertips in a scooping motion clockwise four times and then counterclockwise four times.**
   - Differentiate fingertips from wrist rotating.
   - This allows you to sense the interplay to the forearm more clearly.
   - Notice if your elbows are drooping down.
   - Lift your elbows so as to sense the interplay between the forearms and the upper arms, allowing you to sense the movement going around the elbow joints.
   - Keep the arms below chest level to experience the interplay going into the chest and upper back muscles.
   - Adjust the height of each arm incrementally by lowering the whole arm and bringing it slightly forward to sense the interplay between fingertips and upper torso around the shoulder joint.
   - Keep adjusting the height of each arm until it is just right; that is, until movement goes from one part to the next.
9. **Using the upper chest and upper back muscles, lift the right shoulder from beneath the underarm. Repeat with the left four times.**
   - Do the same with both shoulders four times.

- Lower the arms and bring them forward to sense that the motion of the muscles is lifting the shoulders.

10. Rotate the chest and upper back muscles clockwise four times and then counterclockwise four times.

- End this sequence by lifting your arms above your head and down to the sides of your thighs four times.

  The whole arm sequence exercises the muscles around your lungs to facilitate bigger breaths and allow you to sense the channeling of motion through the torso into the fourth-toe line of the feet,
- Repetition of these fifteen exercises will inevitably increase your flexibility, alignment, and suspension.
- You will find that the interplay will elicit the metaphor of wings in flight in their clockwise rotation and the rolling surf in their counterclockwise rotation.
- The clearer the interplay of muscles, the more readily will the sense of space and the sense of time come to your consciousness.

What is most important is that what you feel about these metaphoric evocations will surface without thought, like a passing breeze. This is the most remarkable outcome of this work!

I have witnessed this process with adults with such a variety of ages and skills over the last fifteen years, that I have hypothesized a relationship between the intrapsychic flow of feelings and the interplay of muscles as irrefutable.

It is a thing to be experienced. Explanations do not easily compute for most people who are used to control and memory as a relationship to the body.

ON YOUR OWN

I could continue to detail all of the exercises, but, as you might already be feeling, it is tiring!

What I have described will help you understand how thoughtfully you need to work to truly and individually realign your musculature. This awareness of the mechanics of motion moving from muscles to muscles will spare you from all sorts of aches and pains that, if left unattended, result in the need for serious and undesirable medical interventions.

Don't hesitate to exercise this subjectively, regardless of whether you do yoga, ballet, modern dance, Afro-Cuban dance, jazz, tai chi, aerobics, or calisthenics, or work out on machines in a gym. Just tell the instructor what you are paying attention to. They will usually support your growing sensitivity to process.

But don't let anybody push you around! The focus of instructors, as I have pointed out, is on the ideal forms of their discipline, and usually does not have anything to do with the way your body needs to work or how you perceive what is happening. *Only you can protect yourself.*

Bringing your attention to the interplay of muscles, to incremental adjustments, and to the symmetry of sensation is not only your best defense against injury; it is also an approach for which you already have all of the necessary means to actuate. You do not have to imagine, conceptualize, or fantasize; just learn to sense what is working, what has to work to do anything with the body, to feel anything through the body.

DON'T GIVE UP

Every incremental adjustment, regardless of how small it may be, improves your alignment and your awareness.

Your sensitivity to the perception of the interplay of muscles is your personal journey into the feeling body.

INTO THE FEELING BODY: THE EVANESCENCE OF THE BODY/MIND SPLIT

I have always tried to render inner feelings through the mobility of the muscles.

Auguste Rodin

PSYCHOLOGICAL, NOT ACTUAL

I have tried to show how psychological most relationships to the body and movement are. The muscles, through which movement happens—through which movement *has to happen*—are experienced as in the service of the wishing, protecting, or anticipating mind. The psychological attachments to the music vary, between instantaneously joining and/or treating it as a demanding annoyance to get away from.

The actuality and simplicity of motion through the interplay of muscles took me many years to appreciate and accept. I was blindly caught up in expelling emotional pain, which I equated with physical tension. I didn't connect my physical tension with conflicted emotions. What was unavoidable was the physical tension within me that demanded mastering the movement skills to control and channel through the body, as some people believe they can do through their minds.

I fell in love with my passion! It took many years for me to understand that my passion was a constant turning into myself that kept reinforcing the tension, no matter how creative I was in choreographing, performing, acting, and directing. Passion was a banner word with a positive spin, a way of talking about the urgency of conflicted feelings that covered up an intangible longing for intimacy.

THE SPLIT

What was split off was my thinking that tension is something to get rid of—whether in the mind or the body. I thought that mastery and control put me in charge of the tension. At another point, I thought that "letting go," allowing the body to totally relax would totally get rid of the tension. When I tried that passive approach, I didn't feel like dancing. The energy of intimacy dissolved into a murky puddle. To dance I had to switch gears and make a decision to dance with relaxation. It just didn't feel right. The split continued.

I realized that I didn't want to get rid of the tension of emotions. I had to find a way to experience feelings that wasn't based on expelling or being received.

TEACHING

I was fortunate that in teaching creative movement, with its improvisational core, I could witness over and over again how children and adults allow what is intimate to come through or how they disconnect to cover up the vulnerability of intimacy. This good fortune allowed me to focus on the process of motion: from exploring the tensions within the boundaries of form, to exploring the gestures and impulses that inform form, to investigating the various canvasses of space and time through which forms emerge and define.

I kept watching movement coming together and falling apart. Inevitably, the fact that motion happens through muscles loomed larger and clearer. How muscles connect and how they are experienced became more important than what comes out or the meaning assigned to them or conjectured about. The process of motion—what sustains and supports it, how it organically evolves, and how it is cut off—became the more helpful aspect to pay attention to and teach.

MASS, WEIGHT, MUSCLES

I kept trying to put what I was observing and experiencing into my engineering/physics-based way of thinking to give it a validation that wasn't just subjective and corroborated by the class members.

Mass is what evolution organizes into nerves, muscles, bones, organs, and so on. Mass has weight, and the muscles are the conduits through which the weight of our bodies transfers as we move. Weight is what the vestibular (balance) system is constantly monitoring, telling muscles throughout the body how to shift instantaneously for support. It is a system that is involved with safety, with survival. It is not a system that cares about intimacy.

Our muscles obey—if they haven't become too rigidly patterned to respond. The stiff body is the pain body of fear. It isn't a fear of the moment; it is a permanent fear woven into the muscles. Maybe it is a defense against the vulnerability of intimacy in which the boundaries of safety are permeable and therefore potentially dangerous.

MOVEMENT AND FEAR

As everyone knows, moving is important. People think of movement as the antidote to stiffening, the unconscious and conscious by-product of fear. I believe that this is why muscles are commonly thought of in terms of flexibility and strength. The poles of strength and flexibility are common determinants of exercise programs.

THE CONTRADICTION

Most people think of support as strength—an erect spine and tight muscles. But flexibility should flow! Isn't this a contradiction? Does one have to develop enough control to be flexible? Or, how can flexibility work and be cohesive?

We marvel at the flexibility of the Olympic skater who has worked out this seemingly contradictory combination. The usual back-story video footage shows them as passionately, obsessively repeating certain moves until idea and execution come together. What we hear from these individuals has nothing to do with the actual process; rather it is a reiteration of passion, discipline, commitment, and gratitude to their coach and parents who supported them.

THE PROCESS

The development of our postural strength has always been in relationship to the ground, not simply our contractive muscular strength. Without the earth we would be, like the famous Rene Magritte's surreal painting *Golconde*, erect, fully suited men with bowler hats, falling through space like raindrops. The ground has always been our basic support!

Infants and toddlers live with the ground, use the ground, but come to believe that it is their muscular contractions, their strength that turns them over, helps them to sit, to stand. Eventually, they will think of contractions as their will, their determination. Their belief is not completely delusional; they are not totally wrong. It is age appropriate to think that they are responsible for what happens that testifies to their egocentricity. The ground is so utterly taken for granted that it isn't considered.

CONTACT, THE GROUND

This understanding of the ground support led to shifting my sense of the body as an object in space to focusing on the weight of the body, and the solid contact of the fourth-toe line of the feet. I had gotten so used to thinking of my body in space, floating in it as if space were empty, or carving it out to cut through it as if it were filled. I never thought about the ground as the support for my weight, channeled through the muscles. I realize in retrospect that I functioned with the unquestioned notion that my support was totally internal, a visualized, imaged alignment of desire, of intentions. A magical body!

AN OBJECT IN SPACE

My experience tells me that most of us relate, unconsciously, to the body, to our support in this way, as if it were all posture, appearance, which we care or do not care about. Conceiving of the self as an object in space is looking at our bodies through the eyes of others. It may start with a mother's gaze, but it comes around to our souls, removed from the actuality of muscular sensation, let alone muscular connections in relationship with the earth.

✦ *A Case in Point* ✦

This brings to mind several former students who had to contend with undeniable physical issues: blindness, rheumatoid arthritis, childhood polio. All of them felt the reality of their impairment but looked at their movement from the outside, as something to contend with, and separated themselves from their conditions. They all changed significantly by learning to focus on the musculature coming through the contact with the floor.

The blind woman came in one morning to tell me that she had overheard a young girl on the subway platform say to another, "I couldn't tell she was blind from the way she walked!" The person whose right side was contracted because of polio, leaving him with a shorter leg, told me, "I stopped falling by sensing the fourth-toe placement of my foot on the ground!" The woman with the severe arthritic condition, who was unable to engage her fingertips without having her knuckles pop out, surprisingly let the motion float through her fingers in her improvisation. Seeing the flow of movement through this woman's hands and fingers sent questions racing through my mind: "What happened to the arthritis? How could it suddenly disappear in an improvisation with a focus on the interplay of muscles?"

These are startling examples. But I saw this process happen again and again over a number of years with my adult students. I watched the conflicted tension about intimacy disappear by way of this physical awareness. It convinced me that there is a relationship between the interplay of muscles and unconscious, unthought-of feelings.

A SIMPLE EXPERIMENT

Lift an arm up. You will quickly begin to experience the heaviness of your arm falling down into your shoulder. This is because the weight is not being experienced through the musculature, even though it is clear to you that you are using muscles to lift the arm. Do the same thing while sensing the musculature from the fingertips through the wrist, forearm, elbow, and upper arm, and you will just as quickly sense the lightness of the arm. You will also quickly realize that to continually sense the motion through the muscles causes you to torque the hand and arm very slowly to connect the motion through the muscles. The incremental torques is the interplay of muscles. It is as simple as that! What reads like a painstakingly slow process becomes light and quick with repeated awareness.

I hope that this little experiment will help you to understand how much we tend to experience movement from the outside, from a judgmental perspective, and from a perspective of desires, cut off from a feeling awareness.

THE EVANESCENT TENSION

The intellectual recognition of this disappearance does not diminish the persistent holding of neck and shoulder muscles, the most common complaint of stress and tension. You have to do the physical work of realigning the musculature. You have to establish new messages to your brain that your support is the ground, the contact moving from your feet through your legs and connecting through the pelvic area before going through the torso into your neck and head.

Making use of the initial instructions at the beginning of the book will go a long way toward relaxing your neck and shoulders. The follow-up interplay of muscles exercises will assure a close-to-permanent solution.

INGESTING VERSUS DIGESTING

What I am about to say might strike you as overly dramatic. However, poets and seasoned psychoanalysts will consider this seriously. The experiment of the arm falling into the body is, metaphorically, a form of ingesting, eating the self, swallowing one's actions. It may seem bizarre to describe it as the ingesting mind, a psychological form of cannibalism, a primitive infantile pattern of possessiveness. But consider that the sensory experience of the gesture, let alone the feeling that emanates, is unwittingly bitten off as the mind chews on the meaning of the action. When the mind contextualizes—swallows too quickly—digestion is hampered. What remains is judgment without due process.

MOTHER EARTH

The ground is our support. The feet are the point of contact with that support. The fourth-toe line on the sole of the foot is the most solid contact with the ground. The sensation of contact experienced through the rest of the body is the interplay of muscles, a body that requires awareness—*the adequate body.*

INTO THE FEELING BODY

The sensation of contact experienced through the interplay of muscles is the resolution of the mind-body split. Both physical and emotional imitations, undertaken with the constant awareness of the contact to the floor, change the muscular process throughout the body. *Kinesthetic awareness* is based on how the brain registers the solid support of the feet. The muscular resistance is not something to get rid off, but a winding path to be followed. It will suspend the weight of the body mass through the muscles, which is easily carried and at times will totally disappear. It is a process that is inclusive of all the other functions of our marvelous mind and heart.

With the interplay of muscles, I found the physical resolution to the tension I had so desperately tried to get rid off by control, by thinking that if I understood it would go away. As if I could make life go away! I found a process that allowed me to digest and metabolize the world around and within me.

I joined the constraints of exercise work to the freedom of improvisation.

Mastery of the body was now based on personal sensitivity to the subtle torques of muscles that facilitate the sensation of contact, which is to be experienced through the whole body. How each person perceives this process is more important than what is imagined, desired, expected, or demanded.

This personal directive results in the evocation of feelings coming through the dance that are unexpected and may not even register on a conscious level. There is a visually apparent organic connection in the phrasing of the improvisation. For those of us watching the individual dancing, the emotional evocation is as palpable as the break of day. Our attention is always riveted. The dancer does not know what will be expressed. What comes through is an organic flow of whatever is going on for the person at that moment. It remains an amazing surprise!

Everything I have ever attempted in the course of these fifty-plus years fits. This process is totally available for all of us. It is nature's framework asking for our awareness.

THE NOW OF EVERYTHING AND YOU

The constancy of the interplay of muscles is the *now*. Contact has to be established each time anew by each one of us. The interplay is the now of attachment, the now of memory, the now of control. The interplay is consciousness, in the simplest terms. It is the transformative junction where body and mind become feelings.

AFTERWORD

Whatever we are feeling on the most unconscious level comes out easily and automatically when we consciously experience the interplay of muscles. Sensing the floor rising through the contact with your feet, resonating through the tactile musculature to the tip of your fingers and head, continually passing throughout, is living fully in the kinesthetic body. The fullness of this awareness is inclusive of everything else that happens in the mind.

The realization that we all have a dynamic system that facilitates this accessibility to our unconscious, to our unthought-of feelings, seems unbelievable when we consider how much our thoughts have a way of becoming convoluted, how conflicted communications in relationships can become, and how arduous descriptions and explanations are when the clarity of feelings don't support these processes.

I have described in a sequential way the continuity of sensation from the soles of the feet touching the floor and up through the musculature. However, once the totality of muscular resonance is sensed, sequence is no longer needed; the conscious mind surprisingly disappears. If you lose the kinesthetic resonance, you can always return to the contact with the ground as the constant base that will never fail you. It is the wholeness that stays alive regardless of what part of the body moves or how fast or slow a movement happens—or whether you move at all.

Every effort to experience the interplay of muscles continually realigns the body through the personal incremental torque of muscles, changing patterns of pain, stress, and repression, while continually enlivening the natural process of our feeling selves. You will be constantly and surprisingly rewarded.

APPENDIX

- 72 percent of Americans say that they do not exercise because of foot pain.[10]
- Thirteen million visits were made to physicians' offices in 2000 due to foot and ankle problems.[11]
- Approximately twelve million visits were made to physicians due to knee problems in 2006.[12]
- Approximately twenty-one million physician visits were made for back problems in 2006, including more than eight million for lower back issues.[13]
- In 2006 musculoskeletal symptoms were the number-two reason for physician visits, with over 132 million visits.[14]
- Musculoskeletal conditions include injuries to bones, joints, muscles, ligaments, and tendons.[15]

---

10 American Podiatric Medical Association, apma.org/2011 feet survey
11 American Podiatric Medical Association, apma.org/2011 feet survey
12 American Podiatric Medical Association, apma.org/2011 feet survey
13 National Ambulatory Medical Care Survey 1998-2006, data obtained from U.S. Department of Health and Human Services Center for Disease Control and Prevention; National Center for Health Statistics, last reviewed and updated, May 2009
14 National Ambulatory Medical Care Survey 1995-2006, data obtained from U.S. Department of Health and Human Services Center for Disease control and Prevention; National Center for Health Statistics, last reviewed and updated, May 2009
15 U.S. Bone and Joint Decade: The Burden of Musculoskeletal Diseases in the U.S., American Academy of Orthopaedic Surgeons, 2008 http//report.nih.gov/NIHfactsheets/ViewFacySheet.aspx

- The average person takes between eight thousand and ten thousand steps per day.[16]
- Mind-body medicine focuses on: the interactions among the brain, the rest of the body, and behavior; the ways in which emotional, mental, social, spiritual, experiential and behavioral factors can directly affect health.[17]

---

16 U.S. Bone and Joint Decade: The Burden of Musculoskeletal Diseases in the U.S., American Academy of Orthopaedic Surgeons, 2008
17 Foot.Com tm www.foot.com/info/info_foot_facts.jsp
15 http//report.nih.gov/NIHfactsheets/ViewFactSheet.aspx

GLOSSARY

Affect: a word used in psychology for feelings.

Creative movement: an approach to dance education that uses exercises, exploring the elements of dance through improvisations to enhance a more subjective experience.

Incremental: measured, very small changes.

Intellectualizing defense: mostly unconscious ways to abort the feeling experience.

Isadora Duncan: an internationally celebrated interpretive dancer of the early 1900s, known for dancing naked, covered only by a diaphanous fabric; known as the mother of modern dance.

Martha Graham: one of the principal pioneering choreographers of the modern dance movement, as influential in the dance as Picasso was in art.

Muscle tonus: refers to the variation in muscular contraction, altering tension of the muscles and qualities of movement, such as soft, hard, and so on.

Point of resistance: the end of a muscle stretching out just so far and no further; the end of an eccentric contraction.

Suspension: distributing effort throughout the rest of the body's musculature, in contrast to rigid skeletal balance.

Swivel: pivoting, as in moving the toes without moving the heel; pivoting the toes in toward the center of the body without moving the heel.

Symmetry: perceiving the same sensation on both sides, requiring personal adjustments.

Weight: sensing the mass of the body; a generalized way of relaxing the muscles; not in regard to numbers on a scale.

ABOUT THE AUTHOR

Mr. Wiener's discoveries in 1959 led to his founding the School for Creative Movement (1962–1992), with over 350 students (more than 200 children aged three to fifteen and 150 adults), movement for actors, teacher training, and summer workshops for students from around the world. Private and group movement therapy began in 1978, and private psychotherapy followed within two years. Mr. Wiener was certified as a psychoanalyst in 1991.

Wiener directed and choreographed more than thirty productions, including the world premiers of Martin Buber's "Elijah," and I. B. Singer's "Gimpel the Fool." He also acted with the Yiddish Folksbiene Theatre in 1963 and '64 and was a featured actor in a film by Bruce Davidson, *Isaac Bashevis Singer's Nightmare and Mrs. Pupko's Beard* (1973). He danced and choreographed for many years (1956–66) and was featured in a *New York Times* magazine article by Anatole Broyard, "It's Your Move." (December 17, 1978). Wiener conducted workshops for Columbia University, Syracuse University, the Toledo Museum of Art, psychoanalytic institutes, the National Psychological Association for Psychoanalysis, and conference presentations for the American Dance Therapy Association, Humanistic Psychology, the National Association for the Advancement of Psychoanalysis, the Institute for Expressive Analysis, and the International Forum for Psychoanalytic Education.

He continues to teach small adult-movement classes, and he maintains a private psychoanalytic and psychotherapy practice in NYC. He lives in Manhattan with his wife, Arlette Thebault Wiener, and their cat, Lili.

www.ingramcontent.com/pod-product-compliance
Lightning Source LLC
Chambersburg PA
CBHW021235280526
45784CB00005B/2107